20,000 Steps

Charity Grant

The Goal

Caught up in a Fitbit® frenzy? You're not alone! In 2014, Fitbit alone sold 11 million devices! That's not counting the step counters sold by Jawbone and Nike, or the dozens of step counting smart phone apps.

And it works! The Fitbit company reports that Fitbit wearers take on average 43% more steps ([1]). Little wonder that companies across the United States are offering Fitbits and similar devices to employees as part of Wellness programs or that Fitbit groups are springing up across towns.

While the urban myth pushes 10,000 steps a day to a healthier you, weight loss gurus recommend at least 20,000 steps to rev up your metabolism and help to walk the pounds off.

Need help getting to 20K steps? Read on!

This little book provides 20 easy changes to add steps to your day. Use these hacks and if you don't hit 20,000 steps by the 11 o'clock news, I will personally come to your house and walk in circles around your dining room wearing your Fitbit® until both of us turn into pumpkins.

Just kidding. Although, not about walking in circles around the dining room at 11 pm. Trust me, I've been there. Luckily, there are easier ways to add steps to your day. Read on!

1. Walk Early

If you're itching to up your steps, try stepping up first thing in the morning by setting aside time for a 15-minute walk before breakfast.

Since the average person takes 2,000 steps per mile ([2]) and walks around 3 miles per hour, this will add around 1,500 steps to your daily total.

It'll also help if you're trying to lose weight. A 2010 study by Belgian researchers ([3]) found that exercising first thing in the morning, before eating, can help subjects to lose weight.

Sort of. What they actually found was that subjects who exercised regularly in the morning could eat 30% more calories and not gain any weight. So while they didn't technically prove that you could lose weight by NOT adding that 30% more calories, that's certainly a logical assumption. If nothing else, adding a short walk before breakfast means that you can go ahead and add cheese to that omelet with less guilt!

2. Walk Late

... and not just in circles around your dining room!

Not everyone is a morning person. Some of us perform better when we're actually awake. If you're also a night owl, take heart. Night owls are fun loving, seem to be more creative, and may even have a higher IQ than their morning person counterparts (4).

So if you'd rather add your steps at night, go for it! In fact, exercising at night has several advantages over morning steps. First, you don't need to get to work or school so you can take your time and really enjoy your stroll. Instead of cramming a 15-minute walk between showering and breakfast, you can take a leisurely 30- to 45-minute stroll around your neighborhood. Heck – you might even get to know some of your neighbors!

Second, you'll probably sleep better. I realize that sounds counterintuitive. According to the *Old Housewives' Medical Compendium* (which sadly exists only in the popular consciousness, not in print), exercising at night is going to keep you awake. However, that's not what the scientific literature says. A 2011 study by Finnish sleep researcher Tero Myllymäki (5) had subjects exercise vigorously for 35 minutes right before bed. The verdict? Those who exercised slept just as well as those who didn't. Later polling data from the National Sleep Foundation found that exercising at night – or really any time at all during the day – actually improves sleep quality. An overwhelming majority (83%) of the 1,000 people they polled in their 2013 Sleep in America® Poll (6) reported sleeping better on days they exercised. The time of day at which they exercised had no effect.

So if your life is better suited to moonlight strolls than predawn jogs, by all means go for it. A 30- to 45-minute evening stroll will add 6,000 to 9,000 steps to your daily total.

3. Pace

Ever since Dr. Levine of the Mayo Clinic popularized the phrase "Sitting is the New Smoking" [7], fidgeting and pacing have gained new respectability. Why? Because the numbers are pretty scary. A 2010 study by the American Cancer Society [8] followed almost 70,000 women for 14 years. Women who sat for six hours a day or more were 94% more likely to die during that 14 years than women who sat for less than three hours a day. If six hours sounds like a lot of sitting to you, remember that that's about a standard day job without an evening of Netflix to follow!

If the death statistics don't make you nervous enough to pace, consider this – people who fidget tend to be naturally lean because they rack up on average 350 extra calories a day. That's a McDonald's cheeseburger with enough calories left over for a handful of fries. Or – if you'd like a little more bang for your calories – that's a Granny Smith apple (80 calories), a Florida navel orange (69 calories), two cups of mixed baby greens (10 calories), one Ritz® cracker (16 calories), two pitted Kalamata olives (18 calories), an entire cooked zucchini (29 calories), one large Kosher dill pickle spear (16 calories), a cup of chopped celery (16 calories), a hardboiled egg (70 calories), eight blueberries (14 calories), and four cherry tomatoes (12 calories). While that would make an odd meal, it is exactly 350 calories. And truthfully, you could probably throw in an extra egg just on the calories you'll accumulate pacing to and from the fridge to retrieve all that food.

So, let's assume you've decided to add pacing to your daily step routine. How many steps can you actually accumulate by pacing?

Quite some time ago, our friend Dr. Levine did some quantification of pacing behaviors. Basically, as part of considering how fidgeting in general affected health, they needed to know how much it is, on average, that fidgeters actually fidget. That's about two hours (9). The thin fidgeters in their study were seated, on average, two hours a day less than their obese colleagues. I'm going to go out on a limb here and assume that if those fidgeters were NOT sitting for an extra two hours per day that they weren't spending those hours standing in place, posed like little Greek statues. So, if we assume they were walking between 60 and 90 minutes of that 120 minutes, that's an extra 6,000 to 9,000 steps a day for pacing.

4. Circle The Kitchen

If you're at home during the day, you probably spend at least two hours of your day in the kitchen. Even if you work outside the home or attend school, you still probably prepare dinner at home and that takes time. A surprising amount of time based on the research by nutrition experts. Overall, women spend about 65 minutes ([10]) per day cooking. That includes time for both preparation and clean up. If you've cooked much, you also know that it includes some intermittent downtime. You know, waiting for the oven to preheat. Watching water boil. That type of thing. Little time killers in which you're not really doing anything but you don't really have enough time to do something else. Perfect pacing opportunities.

Obviously, down time during cooking will vary greatly depending on what it is you're making. There's far more downtime in baking bread (oven preheating, raising time, etc.) than there is in microwaving TV dinners. So let's pick a rather conservative number and say that between five and 15 percent – that is, from three to 10 minutes – of your cooking time is total downtime that you can spend walking in circles around the edges of your kitchen. That adds another 300 to 1,000 steps to your daily total.

5. Walk A Dog

If you don't already have a dog, you're probably thinking, "She's gotta be kidding." And you're right. Sort of.

Dogs are smelly, time consuming, annoying, all around little pain in the butts. Believe me, I know. I own a mutt myself. She's half Australian shepherd, half Chow, and 100% nuisance. BUT she's also my strongest ally in getting fit.

Before you balk at this one, consider the research. According to a study of 3,000 dog owners by esure pet insurance, "the average person walks their dog for 8 hours and 54 minutes a week, covering just under 36 miles in the process, " a habit that adds up to nearly 24,000 miles during the dog's lifetime (11). In steps? That's an astounding 47 million steps over the average dog's lifetime of 12.8 years. Not thinking that far ahead? Breaking that total down gives you close to four million steps per year (3,744,000), or around ten thousand steps a day. Assuming that average falls into the middle of the range, that puts dog walking at an additional 5,000 to 15,000 steps a day.

In addition to their step value, dogs impact walking in numerous ways:

- Dog owners are 62% more likely to walk for leisure than people who don't own pets.

  One California study ([12]) found that dog owners walked 19 minutes per week more than non-pet owners. That's an extra 271 steps per day.

- Dog owners get an extra hour of walking in per week.

  Sometimes. That's assuming that you actually walk your dog. Surprisingly, a full third of dogs are not walked ([13]). If your dog does get his walks, you'll accumulate a full hour of walking per week MORE than the owners of those poor dogs who don't get walks. That is, of course, assuming that you walk Rover yourself. If you use a service, those extra 6,000 steps go to your dog walker.

- Walking with a dog can be even better for you than walking with a person.

  Strange as it sounds, this is especially true for the elderly. A Missouri study of residents at an assisted living facility had some of them walk with a friend or spouse while others went to a local animal shelter and picked a dog to walk ([14]). Over the 12-week study, walking speed increased only 4% among residents walking with a human companion. The dog walkers, on the other hand, were walking 28% faster. I'm not sure how to interpret that. I have to wonder if the human walkers might have been stopping to gossip. Or if the dogs being walked were just dragging those poor old people along, as my own dog is prone to do quite frequently. Regardless, improving speed is still a great thing. Assuming that you walk at an average pace now, upping your speed by 28% would give you an extra 1,680 steps an hour!

- You don't have to own the dog!

That's according to a different study by the same researcher who looked at nursing home residents and dog walking, Rebecca Johnson, RN, PhD. (I guess that makes her Dr. Nurse?) Johnson also looked at dog walking among public housing residents who didn't actually own dogs. While the resulting paper didn't say how many steps the study participants racked up with their "loaner" dogs (borrowed from an animal shelter), it did say that they lost on average 14.4 pounds over the 50-week study ([15]).

No guarantee of weight loss, of course. As Johnson points out in her book, *Walk a Hound, Lose a Pound* ([16]), not only are 70% of Americans overweight – so are 50% of their dogs.

6. Pick A Show

The Nielson people report that American adults spend 36 hours a week watching television ([17]). And that's just traditional TV. Add in streaming services and the number jumps even higher.

Clearly, you can't walk for 36 hours a week without burning yourself out. But you can select just one show per day and opt to walk during that show.

How? There are two methods for walking a TV show:

- Commercials only pacing

  If you're watching traditional television, you're watching a lot of commercials.

  How many commercials? If you're watching broadcast television, you can expect 14 minutes and 15 seconds of commercial ads per hour. On cable, there are even more ads – 15 minutes and 38 seconds worth per hour. ([18])

  Let's take the average, almost exactly 15 minutes. In 15 minutes, you can pace around your living room to the tune of about 1,500 steps.

- Total episode walking

For cord cutters, commercial watching isn't an option. If you have cut the cord, or if you're just highly motivated, you can choose to walk for an entire episode and not just the commercials. At that point, pacing around the coffee table isn't terribly practical. The best way to walk an entire show is to do so on a treadmill. If you belong to a gym, or happen to have a treadmill at home, go for it! You'll probably want to start with a half-hour show and work your way up. That means you'll need to start with a sit-com. For some reason, nearly all half-hour shows are sit-coms and nearly all full-hour shows are dramas or police shows. (There's also the hour and a half show ala *Sherlock* [19] but at that point you might as well just watch a full-length movie...)

Walking through a half-hour sitcom earns you 3,000 steps. Unless you Netflix it. In that case, your half-hour sitcom only lasts for 22 minutes since the commercials are removed. But that still adds up to 2,200 steps. And you'll get a few more if you select an older "Classic" show. MASH (20), for example, runs 25 minutes without the commercials instead of 22.

Ambitious enough for that hour-long drama? Give yourself a gold star and 6,000 steps. Unless you stream it of course. You can keep the gold star but you'll only reap 4,200 steps.

If you're setting long term goals, it might be helpful to choose a series to watch and then get into the habit of walking through one episode a day. With any luck, you'll get sucked into the story line which motivate you to keep watching. If your goal is long term, try a series that was on the air for a while. A large part of my recovery from a broken ankle two years ago was walking my way through all 144 episodes of *Buffy the Vampire Slayer* [21]. At 42 minutes per episode (without commercials since it was streamed), that came to just under 605,000 steps.

If you're just starting your more intensive walking, go for a lighter – and shorter – sitcom. *3rd Rock From the Sun* [22], at 133 22-minute episodes, will keep you busy for nearly five months and add a whopping 293 thousand steps to your annual total.

All those options add up to some serious daily numbers. At the very least, you can add 1,500 steps just by pacing the commercials of a half-hour show. Or, you can walk a full-hour show with commercials for 6,000 steps.

About lying

If you choose to download the TV viewing report from Nielson (the 2015 1st Quarter Audience Report), be advised that the Nielson people will insist on scraping demographic data from your request before they let you download a free copy. That is, the request form will demand name, title, company, phone number, etc. If you're uncomfortable with giving out that information, feel free to lie. I found the download worked just fine using my pen name instead of my real name and giving my phone number as 555-1212 (directory information) with a valid area code.

7. Lunchtime Laps

You're walking early, sneaking in that 15-minute walk before breakfast. You're walking late, enjoying that stroll after dinner. What's missing? A workout to go with lunch, of course.

Walking over the lunch hour is a perfect fit for people tied to a desk job if for no other reason than that lunch is often the only time of day they aren't tied to their desks as well.

Assuming that your lunch hour is an hour (oddly, some aren't), you should be able to sneak in a 15- to 20-minute walk. Or, in Fitbit® parlance, another 1,500 to 2,000 steps.

Worried about what your boss might think? Point her to the research. A recent Scandinavian study ([23]) suggested that lunchtime walks may increase productivity. Specifically? Their study, just published in January 2015, found that lunchtime walkers were more enthusiastic about their work and felt better able to cope with work problems.

8. Schedule Walking Dates

One of the problems you can encounter in maximizing your steps is that in the process you can minimize your social life. No worries! Just combine the two!

Walking with a friend has two major advantages:

- It's fun catching up with your friends on a regularly basis.
- Because it's fun, you're more likely to follow through and actually take the walks you schedule with a friend.

If your friends are too busy for frequent walks, remember that you don't need to be a monogamous walker. Feel free to walk with several friends! I walk with Kathryn in the early morning on Mondays and Wednesdays, Pat over lunch on Thursday, Sally in the early evening on Tuesday, and Sabrina on Monday afternoon and Saturday morning. If that sounds insane, consider that in a typical week, something comes up that ends up cancelling at least three of those walks. That's how life works these days. But since I've scheduled in so many, I still get to see most friends at least once a week for 30 to 45 minutes.

Don't have enough friends to meet your walking goals? Consider joining a walking group. A meta-analysis published in January 2015 in the *British Journal of Sports Medicine* looked at the safety and efficacy of walking groups for improving fitness. Their assessment? "Walking groups are effective and safe with good adherence and wide-ranging health benefits" ([24]). If you live near a park and/or nature center, consider joining a group that walks in natural settings. A recent study published in *Ecopsychology* says that participating in a nature walking group is good for your mental health.

OK, they actually said, "Group walks in nature were associated with significantly lower depression, perceived stress, and negative affect, as well as enhanced positive affect and mental well-being" ([25]). But they meant, walking in nature is really good for your mental health!

How does this impact your steps? At the low end, a single 30-minute walk with a friend after dinner will add 3,000 steps to your weekly total, averaging out to 429 steps a day. At the high end, if you manage to walk with five friends for 45 minutes each over the course of the week, you'll add an average 3,214 steps per day.

9. Cancel The Paper

If you currently subscribe to home delivery of your local newspaper, consider cancelling that service and instead walking to your nearest convenience store to pick up a copy.

There are 152,794 convenience stores in the United States ([26]). If you don't have one nearby, you can usually purchase a newspaper from a local grocery store or gas station. Select one within a 5-minute walk of your home or office and make it a point to buy the weekday paper every day during the workweek. Even better, hit up your change jar on the way to work and pay for that paper with coins. (After all, that's not "real money" anyway!)

The step impact: Five to 10 minutes of walking roundtrip makes for 500 to 1,000 steps. Even if you buy the paper only on weekdays, the normalized average for the week is still an additional 357 to 714 steps a day.

10. Vacuum Daily

Jessica Fisher, writing for the blog *Life As a Mom*, answers the question of how often you should vacuum by first referencing the oft quoted maxim, "You should vacuum an area as many times per week as the number of people that regularly use that area" ([27]). In our household, that would be twice a week while the kids are away at college.

Obviously, Jessica doesn't own a long-haired dog. I collect enough fur from our half Chow each week to build another dog. Seriously. During nice weather I take her outside to brush so often that we now have Tumbleweeds of Chow fur ambling across our lawn.

Daily vacuuming is helpful not only for removing Chow fur, but for accumulating steps. How many?

That's a good question. While I've been able to find statistical references online for thoroughly ridiculous things, I've not been able to find data on how often, or for how long, the average American vacuums. After an exhaustive database search, I had to resort to the unthinkable and actually drag out my own vacuum cleaner and a stop watch. The verdict? Seven minutes per room. About. While it's possible that you vacuum much more thoroughly or efficiently than that, that's the number I have to work with.

According to the United States Census Bureau, the typical American home has three bedrooms, two baths, and central air ([28]). We won't be vacuuming the air compressor, but I'm going to assume that all three bedrooms are carpeted since bedrooms usually are. I'm also going to assume that the living room and family room are carpeted but the kitchen and bathrooms are not. That makes for five rooms to vacuum at seven minutes a piece, and we'll throw in an extra three minutes for dragging the vacuum cleaner from room to room. That's 38 minutes for a total of 3,800 steps.

Now we make some wild guesses to arrive at our totals. I'm going to assume that no one vacuums less than once a week, and I'll put the maximum (for households with small children, fluffy cats, and Chows) at once a day, even though, in all honesty, there have been days when I've vacuumed my living room three times and still ended up covered in Chow fur. Using these outer limits puts the step range for vacuuming at 543 to 3,800 steps per day.

11. Consider A Walking Desk

With this one insanely expensive and decadent exception, every suggestion that I make in this book can be pulled off at absolutely no cost. This is the one exception. And it is a doozy.

A decent treadmill desk will run you about $1,500 to $2,000. I use a LifeSpan, but there are a number of good options. You'll see them occasionally on Amazon for $800 but those aren't adjustable. So if you're not exactly 5 foot 8; you'll want to take a pass.

In a perfect world, you can talk your employer into investing in treadmill desks as part of the company wellness program. Probably not though. Which means you'll need to consider how much work you do at home to decide whether it's worth the investment.

As a writer, I work about four hours a day. (Lucky me!) Of those, I spend two on the treadmill. I also watch an episode of CSI (a fantastic walking choice now that all 15 seasons – 335 episodes – are being streamed on Hulu! [29]) in the evening.

And I spend about an hour in the morning reading my email and scanning the daily news. That's four hours total on the treadmill.

So far, we've been estimating walking at 6,000 steps per hour because that's assuming a normal walking pace of three miles per hour. Your treadmill desk pace is going to vary wildly depending on what you're doing. For example, I can watch CSI at 3.8 miles per hour, which is actually the maximum speed of my treadmill. I can check my email and surf the web at around 2.5 miles per hour. But I need to slow it down to about 1.5 miles per hour in order to type, which is kind of important with the me-being-a-writer thing.

So for me, the treadmill desk adds about 18,000 steps per "work" day, and I work most often four days a week. That averages out to 10,286 steps per day. If I watched more TV shows on Netflix® and did less typing, I'd get in a lot more steps. But again, that would be somewhat problematic with the me-being-a-writer thing.

If you're not a writer by trade, you'll probably use the walking desk somewhat less. Unless of course you work from home doing transcription, social media marketing, or web research. It's really hard to guess. For now, I'm going to throw out fuzzy numbers and assume that my usage is toward the high end of middle. That gives us a step range of 6,000 to 20,000 steps for adding a walking desk to your collection of office furniture.

12. Think On Your Feet

This comes under the general category of pacing, but there is a distinction. For the most part, I'd like you to consider thinking on your feet at the office.

Ideally, office workers should be on their feet for at least four hours every day. That's to avoid the nasty health effects of a sedentary lifestyle, at least according to a study co-commissioned by Public Health England ([30]). The 2015 study recommends that workers stand for at least two hours a day, working up to four hours of standing.

A simple way to do this is to make it a point to stand and pace while you think. If you actually spend less than two hours thinking in your day job, that's a problem of a different color.

For now, let's assume that you meet the recommendations of the *British Journal of Sports Medicine* and stand and think at the office between two and four hours per day. Sort of. We're going to take the physicians' self-reporting approach and reverse it. You know, where the doctor asks you how much you drink or smoke then writes down twice whatever you say. In terms of exercise, the approach is to halve the self-reported number. What s/he's doing is correcting for the natural inclination people have to want to make themselves look better than they are. It's like TV watching. You know why the Nielson people started handing out those silly boxes that automatically track what people watch? Because people lie. Not just to keep their favorite shows from being cancelled, although there is a bit of that. Mostly they lie to avoid embarrassing themselves by claiming to watch a lot more "classy" documentaries and PBS specials and a lot fewer "trashy" reality shows than they actually do. It's human nature. The same thing happens when people are asked about their exercise habits. So we're going to assume that office workers expected to walk two to four hours a day are actually going to walk one to two hours a day and then fudge a bit when reporting this behavior to their employers.

In steps? That would be 6,000 to 12,000 steps during the workweek. Averaged over seven days (unless you're planning to work 24/7 which would be bad on a number of other levels), that comes to 4,286 to 8,571 steps per day.

13. Make Bedtime Rounds

The last time you left for an out of town vacation, how many times did you circle your house, compulsively checking that you'd locked all the doors, closed all the windows, and turned off the lights and appliances you meant to leave off for the duration? Probably at least three. Clearly, you wouldn't want to do that every night. Our goal here is to sneak extra steps into your day, not load up on new obsessive behaviors for your therapist to sort out.

However, you could do a shorter, slightly less OCD version of bedtime rounds. Once around the house, stopping in each room to check windows, lock doors, and turn off the lights. Granted this isn't a lot of steps, but since we're adding a few steps here and there (and everywhere!), you'll see quickly that those little bits really add up. In fact, if you jumped to the *Tallying It Up* chapter, you'd see that at this point in the book – even without those bedtime rounds – you've already added over 20,000 steps to your day just by following the first 12 recommendations! But, back to *this* chapter...

The typical American home has three bedrooms, two baths, a kitchen, a separate dining room, and a separate garage or carport. Oddly, the majority don't have two or more living rooms (for example, family rooms, rec rooms), which I would have expected.

Since the census data doesn't report the average size of each of those typical rooms, I'm going to make a wild guess and assume that all rooms are the size of my dining room. There are a couple of advantages to this. One is that it makes for a nice easy number to work with. The other, more important factor, is that I already know how many steps it takes to walk around my dining room, having circled that room more times than I care to admit when the 11 o'clock news was ending and I still hadn't made my step goal for the day. The magic number? 23 steps. That would be circling the dining room table, in and out the kitchen and hall doors, but not stopping to touch the corners or anything too *Monk* like ([31]). [If you haven't seen it, *Monk* is a detective show about an obsessive compulsive police detective who spends much of his time touching trees. Surprisingly entertaining! It would be well worth a try if you need to pick a new TV show to walk along to.]

And again, back to this chapter. Let's assume that 23 steps around the room is your average size. That's probably a fair guess since my dining room is much bigger than most bathrooms but much smaller than most living rooms. And we're also going to assume that your bedtime routine includes checking only one of the bedrooms – yours. You really don't want to wake up your kids every night as you make the bedtime rounds, but we will throw in another 30 steps so you can walk down the hall and peek into the kids' bedrooms. The total? That's 23 steps each for five rooms (115 steps) and another 30 steps for the hall for a total of 145 steps. If you live in a McMansion, you can double that to 290 steps. Sound like nothing? Imagine it over the course of a year. Just 145 steps a day becomes 53,000 steps or three hours of walking. Since most people walk around a 20-minute mile, that corresponds to nine miles of walking. Would it take you three years to finish a marathon at this pace? Well, yes. But we can't all finish first, can we?

14. Take Out The Recycling

Emptying your recycling containers is one more excuse to wander around your house from room to room, leaving little clean spots in your wake and accumulating steps in the process.

If you live in apartment building with a dumpster for recyclables, this is a task you can do daily. While you're at it, go ahead and take the trash out as well. Emptying your trash daily will keep it small, so you'll be able to reuse those free grocery store plastic bags instead of buying trash bags. It'll also help to minimize the creepy crawlies. In fact, one of the top recommendations to eliminate German cockroach infestations is to either remove indoor trash cans, or keep them emptied (32). That would apply to recycling as well. In addition to having the purported ability to survive a nuclear war, roaches can live for ages on nothing but empty cardboard boxes and paper bags. Really. They eat them. According to Cornell University's Integrated Pest Management program website, "Roaches eat anything that is organic–even cardboard and the glue that binds books together" (33).

If you live in a standalone dwelling (you know, a regular house!), you can still collect up your recycling every day and store it in your garage or carport to await trash day. Assuming you'll be emptying this recycling at least every few days, go ahead and put small recycling bins in those areas of the house where you're most likely to accumulate recyclables. I think we all have recycling bins around the kitchen for glass bottles, plastic jugs, and paperboard (that flat cardboard used to make cereal boxes). But how about the bathroom? A bathroom recycling bin is useful for empty cardboard toilet paper rolls, plastic shampoo and conditioner bottles, and even the paperboard wrappers for those three-packs of deodorant soap. If you're thinking that you don't have space, don't think large official looking oversized recycling bin. Think tiny wastepaper basket. Remember, you'll be emptying this all the time so you don't want a large bin.

The time and steps required to collect up little recycling baskets and dump that trash into the larger recycling receptacle will depend on whether you live in a little bungalow in the suburbs with an attached car port or a 5th floor walkup apartment in the city. I'm going to guesstimate the range between 150 and 200 steps and assume that you'll take out the recycling between three and seven times a week (at least every other day). That gives you a step range of 450 to 1,400 steps per week or 65 to 200 steps per day.

15. Park Further Away

The trick to accumulating steps by parking further away is to apply this trick to both shopping and employment.

Let's start with shopping. The Time Use Institute reports that on any given day, one out of seven Americans is at the grocery store (34). According to the Food Marketing Institute's 2012 U.S. Grocery Shopper Trends Executive Summary, American shoppers hit the grocery store 2.2 times per week. That's just the grocery mind you – not the Dollar store for paper plates, the Rutter's convenience store for milk without added growth hormones, or Costco for giant packages of paper towels, etc. Those non-grocery store grocery sources are what the industry calls "small formats" although it's really hard to think of that Walmart Supercenter as a small format. For our purposes though, let's consider just the official grocery store trips and round down to twice a week.

In the bizarre trivia department, the average parking space appears to be about eight feet wide. Wikipedia reports a range of 7.5 to 9 feet while noting that the average widths in Dallas, Texas are 7.5 feet for compact cars and 8.5 feet for standard cars (35). Even though there are generally far more "standard" spots than "compact" spots, we're going to average these together and go with eight feet even. While much aligned as a reference source, the truth is that a rather infamous *Nature* study from 2005 found that Wikipedia is almost as accurate as the Encyclopedia Britannica ([36]). For our purposes, Wikipedia really is better because it has the advantage of containing bizarre factoids that fail to interest the Britannicans such as the average width of American parking spaces. If you're fact checking, consider that the Americans with Disabilities act requires handicapped parking spaces to be at least eight feet across with an additional 5-foot access path ([37]). Just eyeballing your average Walmart parking lot, if those handicapped spaces are 13 feet, then eight feet seems about right for the rest of them.

Incidentally, if you'd like the best selection of parking spaces, do your grocery shopping early in the week. While 41 million Americans grocery shop on Saturday, only 29 million head out on Monday or Tuesday ([38]).

Parking at the end of a 20 space row instead of up front will add 144 feet to your walk. (That's eight feet times 18 spaces back. I'm not counting the 19th, because you would have gotten out on the far side of the first space anyway, since that's where the driver's seat is.) The average person has a stride length of

2.5 feet; that's where I got the figure of 2,000 steps per mile that I've been using throughout (39). Using 2.5 feet per "step", that 144 feet of extra walking adds an extra 58 steps in each direction. Assume two grocery trips per week and that's an extra 34 steps per day.

If you're retired, a homemaker, unemployed, or self-employed in the home, that's all you get for this hack. But if you drive to your place of employment, you can park further away at your job as well as your favorite supermarket.

I'm going to assume that your employer is a bit smaller than Whole Foods or the Price Chopper, so you probably can't park 18 spaces further back. But you probably can park five spaces back. Using the same figure of eight feet across each parking space, you can add 13 steps in each direction or 26 steps each workday. If you leave work (by car) to go home for lunch, run errands, etc. you can double that number. Let's assume that you work five days a week and drive home for lunch every day. That gives you a maximum benefit of 71 steps a day for this hack – 37 steps for parking further from your job added to the 34 steps for parking further out in the supermarket parking lot.

16. Launder Slowly

In *The Miracle of Mindfulness*, Buddhist guru Thích Nhất Hạnh discusses the application of mindfulness to everyday tasks like washing the dishes:

"I clean this teapot with the kind of attention I would have were I giving the baby Buddha or Jesus a bath. Nothing should be treated more carefully than anything else." (40)

OK, that's probably a little more existential than you were looking for. Or a little too New Age for your tastes. If so, consider the Christian alternative. In her blog entry for Madonna House, Melanie Murphy also talks about dishwashing as a form of prayer (41).

The basic gist in both philosophies is that being conscious of what you're doing – really, truly conscious of it – can be a form of spiritual practice that soothes your soul.

I'd like you to apply that to laundry. How you ask? By mindfully considering each piece of laundry as it emerges from the dryer. Warm, fresh, inviting. One at a time – that's the really important part – lovingly fold or hang the freshly laundered item and then immediately put it away in the dresser, closet or wardrobe where it belongs.

How much of an impact could this have? Quite a bit. The average family of four does eight loads of laundry per week (42).

What's in a load? That's harder to say. Washing machines hold between six and 18 pounds of clothing per load (43). A pair of adult jeans weighs about three pounds. A man's dress shirt, under one pound. And those risqué ladies G-strings having the approximate style and substance of dental floss seem to have no weight at all. I imagine they'd float off on their own from the washer if they weren't ensnared by the lost socks living under the agitator.

Given the lack of academic data on this topic, I headed off to my own laundry room and just counted items emerging from the dryer. So for my house anyway, there appear to be 15 to 20 items of clothing per load. As a disclaimer, our children are grown now so you won't find any miniature baby socks or baby bibs unless the grandkids are visiting. And the last of those dental floss knickers were swallowed whole by a pair of granny pants sometime in the late 90s. So my baskets may or may not represent the quantity of your laundry. Be that as it may, I'm going to assume an average family with average loads of laundry. That would be 15 to 20 items per load and eight loads per week. I'm also going to assume an absolute minimum average of 15 steps round trip from dryer to closet for each item. For the maximum, we'll assume that your laundry is in the basement and add 20 steps – literally steps in this case – to each trip. What's that get you? At the lower end, 15 items per load in a tiny apartment with only 15 steps from dryer to closet gets you 257 steps a day just putting away the laundry. At the higher end, you get 700 steps a day.

For those of you in larger households or with small children and perpetually running washing machines, you might want to apply this hack to every other load – or at least no more than eight loads per week. After all, we're hoping to soothe your soul – not damage your soles!

At the other end, if you're an empty nester thinking that eight loads a week is far too much, be sure to count the loads of laundry that you actually do. When our last kid left the nest for a freshman dorm, I found that at least initially I was doing more laundry as I caught up with the "annual" washing of blankets, curtains, etc. that had turned into bicentennial events. Our laundry jumped again while I was writing Kitchen Decluttering: 30 Days to Clutter Free! (44) and discovered that my kitchen sink is a festering pool of bacteria. In the category of things you probably wish you didn't know, a recent study found that 89 percent of American and Canadian kitchen towels were contaminated with coliform bacteria and over 25% tested positive for E. coli [45]. That study added an extra load just of tea towels and dishcloths to my weekly washing.

17. Pick The Farthest Potty

You're already added steps by parking your car farther from the grocery store or your job. Have you thought about parking yourself farther from the bathroom? Or, to take a different perspective, what about choosing to walk to the farthest bathroom in your home or office?

Before you laugh too hard, consider that according to the Bladder and Bowel Foundation, people who certainly know their pee, the typical adult urinates between six and seven times per day ([46]). That's on average. You can pee as few as four or as many as 10 times a day and still be within the normal range. [Of course, if you're a woman who's had more than three children or a man over 50 who now knows exactly what a prostate is, you already know that.]

Back to the average, if you're running to the loo six or seven times a day, heading for a farther bathroom can really rack up some steps. Most likely 40 or 50 steps round trip, including 20 actual steps since the farther bathroom in your home or office is very likely to be on a different floor. Using the far ranges of normal, taking those 40 to 50 steps on your four to 10 trips to the bathroom will give you a range of 160 to 500 extra steps a day. This could be one of the few cases where having an overactive bladder works in your favor.

18. Sweep It Up

Sweeping it up is where the hardwood floor owners make up for the steps that they lost in the vacuuming challenge.

If you have a very new or a fairly old house, chances are that you have hardwood floors. In new homes, hardwood floors are a big selling point. Leslie Piper, a consumer housing specialist with Realtor.com, contends that today's buyers expect hardwood and may very well pass on homes with wall-to-wall carpeting instead (47). For older homes, hardwood was actually a requirement. Until the mid-1960s, the U.S. Department of Housing and Urban Development (HUD) wouldn't back the mortgages for homes without hardwood floors (48). Their reasoning was that wood floors contributed to the structural integrity of the home. So if your home was built before the 1960s, there's a strong possibility that what's under your wall-to-wall carpeting is actually real wood and not just a wood subfloor. [Unless of course, it's not. So please don't rip up any carpeting based on my say so!]

Even without hardwood, odds are good that you have tile or linoleum in your kitchen and bathrooms. If you don't, my condolences. When we purchased our home from a lovely family with two toddler boys, the first thing we did was rip out the carpet in the main bathroom and install a nice no-wax vinyl floor. I suspect those boys never once hit their Tinkle Targets (49). Even the subfloor was drenched...

Getting back to our steps, at minimum you'll have the kitchen and the main bathroom to sweep. Add to that sweeping of hardwood floors in the living room and dining room. Broom sweeping takes roughly the same time as vacuuming, seven minutes a room. Those bathrooms will take a lot less though, about four minutes. This puts your step range for this hack at 1,100 steps (sweeping kitchen/main bath only) to 2,400 steps.

19. Walk For A Cause

I have a dear old friend, Edna, who decided years ago to forgo the traditional gym membership and instead participate in charity walks and 5Ks. Her philosophy was that it was cheaper than a gym membership and she was helping out good causes at the same time.

She was right. According to StatisticBrain.com, the average monthly cost of a gym membership (as of April 2015) is $58 ([50]). The typical cost of a charity walk, assuming you don't register at the last minute, is $35. So for almost half the cost of a gym membership, Edna can participate in a different 5K every month.

This got me thinking. I wonder if most people could find enough 5Ks to pull that off? I live in a fairly small town but with a heavy tourist trade, Gettysburg, PA, so I started by looking for 5Ks in the vicinity.

In Gettysburg proper, I found:

- The Spirit of Gettysburg 5K - Sponsored by the YWCA ([51])
- The Hard Cider Run - Sponsored by Hauser Estate Winery, makers of Jack's Hard Cider ([52])

- The Gateway 5K – Held at the opening of the Gettysburg Blue-and-Grey Half Marathon (53)
- The Red, White & Blue 5K Color Run – Sponsored by the Gettysburg Area Recreation Authority (54)
- Anything is PAULssible 5K – Held in memory of Gettysburg College student Paul Detweiler who passed away in 2013 from a cancerous brain tumor (55)

And those were just the 5Ks held in town that I could find in a 15-minute web search. If I extended my search to a drivable area of say 90 minutes in each direction, I could easily do a 5K once or twice every weekend year round, with the possible exception of dead of winter. If you live in a warmer area, you could probably do a different 5K every month year round.

Outside of the added steps and the warm fuzzies you get from helping out a good cause, most 5Ks are just a lot of fun. If you enjoy vibrant colors, you should also check out the many Color Runs. A Color Run is a 5K version of the Hindu Celebration of Colors during the Festival of Holi. Basically, you dress in white and jog along as spectators douse you with colored powders. By the finish line, it's literally a walking rainbow.

5Ks are also favorite fundraisers among zoos. I ran one this past April in North Carolina near my grandchildren. The Greensboro Science Center Tuxedo Trot is an annual 5K held to raise funds for endangered African penguins (56). Scores of participants show up wearing tuxedos or dressed as penguins. I ran (and I do use that term quite loosely!) with my oldest daughter. Similar events are held nationwide, including the Pittsburgh Zoo & Aquarium's ZooZilla 5K (57), the Lehigh Valley Zoo Run Wild for Wildlife Conservation in Pennsylvania (58), Run Wild for the Detroit Zoo in Michigan (59), the Samson Stomp & Romp at the Milwaukee Zoo (60) in Wisconsin, the Jungle Jog at the Seneca Park Zoo (61) in New York, ZooRunRun at the Chicago Zoo (62), ZooRun5K at Zoo Miami (63), and the Cheetah Run 5K at the Cincinnati Zoo (64).

If the cause closest to your heart is say, Heart Disease, and not critters, there's a walk for that too. In 2015, there were 305 HeartWalks nationwide; quite likely one near you (65). I've also seen 5Ks hosted to raise funds and/or awareness for a wide range of other diseases and conditions. Many of these are nationwide. You can Walk to Cure Arthritis (66), Walk to End Alzheimer's (67), join a NAMI Walk to raise awareness of mental illness (68), attend the National Parkinson Foundation's Moving Day® Walk (69), or take the Kidney

Walk (⁷⁰). If you're not keen on ice water, you can even Walk to Defeat ALS (⁷¹).

Don't feel that you need to complete an entire 5K either. Many charity events also include a one mile option. For example, that Seneca Park Zoo run offers the Seneca Park Zoo mile (⁷²) as well as the 5K Jungle Jog.

If the weather isn't accommodating, or the entrance fees are a bit much for your budget, you can also walk for a cause by downloading a free app that converts your miles into donations at no cost to you. One of my favorites is ResQWalk (⁷³). The ResQWalk app raises funds via advertising to users and splits that pool each week between the Animal Rescues that have signed up to receive donations. The percentage that each Animal Rescue gets depends on how many miles their supporters logged. If you want your local shelter to get a bigger check, you walk more. A similar app, Walk for a Dog, is available from WoofTrax (⁷⁴).

Charity Miles (⁷⁵) is another free app that converts your steps into cash for the charity of your choice. While you can select from dozens of charities, the one that spoke to my sense of balance for this app was Soles4Souls (⁷⁶), which provides shoes for the poor.

So how does all this charitable walking affect your step tally? That depends on how often you do it. For our calculations, I'm going to factor in only the 5K events. By all means, make use of the charity walking apps, but you'll probably do that while you're walking with a friend, picking up your cancelled newspaper at the 7/11, or hiking to the produce section from the far outer expanses of the parking lot. The new steps will be just the 5Ks.

For those of you who aren't yet fluent in metric, five kilometers is 3.1 miles or 6,200 steps. Let's assume that you do a minimum of one 5K walk/run per year and a maximum of one 5K walk/run per month. Averaged over the year, that's another 17 to 204 steps per day.

20. Make It A Contest

Amazing, you're already on to the last challenge!

If you're using an actual Fitbit® as opposed to another brand of wearable step counter, you can use the Fitbit Challenges to initiate competitions with friends who are also Fitbit® wearers. These competitions run from a single day to a full week and include the Daily Showdown, Weekend Warrior, Workweek Hustle, and Goal Day. That last one, the one that's not blatantly obvious, can have multiple "winners" since every person who meets their step goal for the day actually "wins".

The rest of the challenges usually go to the most compulsive participant. (The one who's willing to walk circles around her dining room at a quarter to midnight just to pass you up by 40 or 50 steps!)

Up to 10 Fitbit users can participate in any given challenge. And you can participate in multiple challenges at the same time with different people.

It's hard to say how many additional steps you'll earn this way because that depends entirely on how competitive you are. Personally, just joining a competition upped my daily steps by at least 2,000. Even when I didn't have a chance of winning, I didn't want to look like a complete slug and ended up exceeding my step goal as a result. So I'm going to throw out what our household contractor calls a SWAG (silly wild-arsed guess) and attribute another 100 to 2,000 steps a day to some friendly competition.

Do think carefully when you're deciding who to challenge. First, some people are going to wipe the floor with you simply by default. For example, I have a good friend who works nightshift cleaning at a local factory. Her job actually requires her to walk around for the better part of eight hours a night. I just can't compete with those numbers.

You'll also find that some people prevaricate. You know, cheat! I was scanning Friends' Facebook photos the other day when I noticed something odd in a grandkid photo on one of my competitive friend's timelines. Yup – it was a Fitbit. She'd strapped it onto her 2-year-old granddaughter's ankle. If you don't have toddlers, that's like attaching it to a perpetual motion machine. I was toast before that challenge even started.

It also cracked me up for the better part of a week just thinking about it. Which is the point of this book. You really, really need to have fun with it!

Tally It Up

First, I hope you get it by this point that this little book is as tongue-in-cheek as it is practical. If you followed all the steps in this book, you'd be walking pretty much 24/7. Having said that, you really can add a massive number of steps to your daily walking with these ideas. How many? The following chart puts the minimum and maximum step counts from each challenge in one place with a tally at the end. If you rise to every challenge described in this little book, you would add between 30,000 and 80,000 steps to your daily total. Which is ridiculous! Truthfully, no one has time to do everything I've listed. Instead, focus on choosing four or five of the possibilities that tickle your fancy and fit your schedule. Assuming you weren't in a coma when you started reading, that should easily get you to 20,000 steps.

Should you add up your new steps? Uh, no... Have a look at your wrist. The reason you agreed to be banded then released to the wild was to make sure that someone else – or something else in this case – had to count up all your steps!

	Minimum	Maximum
Walk Early	1,500	1,500
Walk Late	3,000	4,500
Pace	6,000	9,000
Circle The Kitchen	300	1,000
Walk a Dog	5,000	15,000
Pick A Show	1,500	6,000
Lunchtime Laps	1,500	2,000
Schedule Walking Dates	429	3,214
Cancel the Paper	357	714
Vacuum Daily	543	3,800
Consider A Walking Desk	6,000	20,000
Think On Your Feet	4,286	8,571
Make Bedtime Rounds	145	290
Take Out The Recycling	65	200
Park Further Away	34	71
Launder Slowly	257	700
Pick the Farthest Potty	160	500
Sweep It Up	1,100	2,400
Walk For A Cause	17	204
Make It A Contest	100	2000
Total	**32,293**	**81,664**

About The Author

My name is Charity Grant. Except, of course, that it isn't.

Charity Grant (as you may have suspected) is a pen name. This isn't because I'm ashamed of my cluttering tendencies and slug-like exercise routine and wish to avoid airing my dirty laundry in public. Nor do I write erotica on the side, which strangely everyone seems to assume when you admit to using a pen name. Nope. No *50 Shades of Fitbit®* for me.

Truth be told, I use a pen name only because my real name is just awful for publishing. It's got 12 characters. Six vowels and six consonants, with a hyphen thrown in for complexity, and ending in an "iy" combination that never appears in basic English. The upshot? No one can pronounce it. And even my best friend can't spell it.

As an author, I'd really like fans to be able to find my works online. That means they need to be able to remember and spell my name. That just wasn't going to happen if I insisted on publishing under my real name. So instead, I selected a pen name that I thought represented me – or at least the "me" I would like to be.

I went for Charity because charity is something that's very important to me. Over the years, my family and I have made volunteering a central part of our family life. Year after year, we've invited our friends to an Easter party to dye eggs for the local soup kitchen. We've walked dogs at the local SPCA. One year, we took kittens to the Alzheimer's ward at a public nursing home on Fridays. Every year, we conscientiously weed our wardrobes and donate the surplus to the Hospital Thrift Shop. In 2008, we collected over a thousand pair of new socks and underwear that we distributed to the local homeless shelter and battered women's shelter. To give you an idea of just how important "charity" is to our family, in 2007, we were awarded the *Heart in Hand Award* for volunteering in the family category by the United Way of Adams County here in Gettysburg, Pennsylvania. Given this history, "Charity" represented the image I chose to present to the outside world far better than my given name, a derivation of Dionysius – the Greek God of wine. Nothing against wine, of course. But I definitely still prefer Charity.

The surname Grant I selected for similar reasons. During my years of working with the local soup kitchen, I wrote numerous successful grant proposals. Because of that, I always associate the word "grant" with gift. That's a nice association. Even better, it's a nice association that's easy to pronounce and almost impossible to misspell!

Hence was born, Charity Grant.

Additional Books By This Author

If you enjoyed this book, please consider reading additional books written by Charity Grant and her fiction writing alter-ego, Jadzia Banks.

Nonfiction

KITCHEN DECLUTTERING: 30 DAYS TO CLUTTER FREE!

Your kitchen may not be the only cluttered room in your house, but it is absolutely the one you need to clean first. Why? Because unless you rely on takeout for three meals a day, and leave the house before drinking your morning coffee, you really can't avoid your kitchen. Luckily, you can whip it into shape in only 30 days. That's rational time, not 1-800-GOT-JUNK showing up and emptying it out time. In only 30 days, spending on average 30 minutes a day, you can transform your kitchen from a disaster to a clutter free zone.

CROWDFUNDING HOMESCHOOL EXPENSES

Unlike public school students, homeschoolers can't rely on state or federal funding. But they can, and sometimes do, take advantage of the relatively new phenomena of crowdfunding to provide funds for everything from field trips to basic curricula.

Fiction

BETTA VIRUS: A JADZIA BANKS SHORT STORY (KINDLE SINGLE)

It was old science, published back in 2011, but the implications intrigued her. Adira wasn't as interested in eliminating fear as she was in generating it. What if instead of removing a healthy fear (like fear of a predator's smell), a similar mechanism could be used to implant an unhealthy fear? Better yet, an overwhelming, anxiety-laden, paralytic fear? Could she generate a Betta fish reaction in humans?

Please Review This Book

As an independent author, I depend on word of mouth and good reviews to sell books. While it would be great if it were otherwise, my current advertising budget is $14.85 plus 259 Yen from a book sale on Amazon's Japan market.

Ah... Scratch the yen. Turns out that at the current exchange rate that will buy me a pack of gum on my next (first?) trip to Tokyo.

If you could post a nice review of this book, I'd really appreciate it.

Sources

Anytime you see a statistic, or health claim, or quotation, it's important to ask yourself – Where did this come from? Is this author quoting valid scientific research? Believing everything that she reads on the Internet? Or simply making it up as she goes?

To help you make that assessment, I've included links to all the sources for information that I've referenced in this book.

Throughout the text, I've hyperlinked the sources for each statistic, adding the full address for every hyperlink as an endnote. If you're reading the print version, you can find those hyperlinked web addresses here.

The note numbers appear throughout the text. Just look up the note number below to find the address of each source.

---

[1] http://www.fitbit.com/about

[2] http://www.thewalkingsite.com/10000steps.html

3 http://www.ncbi.nlm.nih.gov/pubmed/20837645

4 http://personal.lse.ac.uk/kanazawa/pdfs/paid2009.pdf

5 http://www.ncbi.nlm.nih.gov/pubmed/20673290

6
http://sleepfoundation.org/sites/default/files/RPT336%20Su
mmary%20of%20Findings%2002%2020%202013.pdf

7 http://www.juststand.org/tabid/674/default.aspx

8 http://aje.oxfordjournals.org/content/172/4/419.abstract

9 http://www.sciencemag.org/content/307/5709/584.short.
This particular article is free to read, however you will need to
create a free account at *Science* magazine in order to access it.

10 http://www.ncbi.nlm.nih.gov/pmc/articles/PMC3639863/

11
http://www.esure.com/media_centre/archive/doggy_mileage
.html

12 http://www.ncbi.nlm.nih.gov/pubmed/18382031

13

http://www.americankinesiology.org/AcuCustom/Sitename/Documents/DocumentItem/15_reeves_JPAH_2009_0013a.pdf

14 http://rechai.missouri.edu/previous-research/

15 http://www.ncbi.nlm.nih.gov/pubmed/20651066

16 http://www.amazon.com/Walk-Hound-Lose-Pound-Human-Animal-ebook/dp/B005146XAQ

17 http://www.nielsen.com/us/en/insights/reports/2015/the-total-audience-report-q1-2015.html This report is free but they will require that you enter identifying information in the request form. Feel free to identify someone else.

18

http://www.nielsen.com/us/en/insights/news/2014/advertising-and-audiences-making-ad-dollars-make-sense.html

19 http://www.imdb.com/title/tt1475582/

20 http://www.imdb.com/title/tt0068098/

[21] http://www.imdb.com/title/tt0118276/

[22] http://www.imdb.com/title/tt0115082/

[23] http://www.ncbi.nlm.nih.gov/pubmed/25559067

[24] http://bjsm.bmj.com/content/early/2014/12/19/bjsports-2014-094157.full

[25]

http://online.liebertpub.com/doi/abs/10.1089/eco.2014.0027 . This article is currently available only to paid subscribers (mostly libraries) or to researchers willing to pay the $134 pay per view fee to read the entire article. I don't imagine you'll want to do that. But I'm leaving the link in anyway because article accessibility changes quickly. Most academic journals have a rolling embargo by which you have to pay for the most recent articles but you can read the older articles for free. In most cases, the embargo period ranges from six months to two years. So it's entirely possible that this article will be free by the time some readers click on this link.

[26] http://www.nacsonline.com/asknacs/pages/how-many-convenience-stores-are-there-in-the-united-states.aspx

27 http://lifeasmom.com/2010/08/how-often-should-you-vacuum.html

28

http://factfinder.census.gov/faces/tableservices/jsf/pages/productview.xhtml?pid=AHS_2013_C02AH&prodType=table

29 http://www.hulu.com/csi-crime-scene-investigation

30 http://bjsm.bmj.com/content/early/2015/06/30/bjsports-2015-094618. Like the earlier *Ecopsychology* article, this particular paper is currently available only on pay-per-view. While it is considerably cheaper than *Ecopsychology*, at $37 versus $134, the *British Journal of Sports Medicine* does their pay-per-view by the day. Rather like renting a movie on Amazon except for the part where what you get is a fairly boring jargon filled medical paper instead of a nice romance or a wicked action film. So if you go this route, remember to read or print quickly before your 24-hour access expires.

31 http://www.imdb.com/title/tt0312172/

32 http://www.doyourownpestcontrol.com/german.htm

33 http://nysipm.cornell.edu/publications/roach/think.asp

34

http://timeuseinstitute.org/Grocery%20White%20Paper%20
2008.pdf

35

https://en.wikipedia.org/wiki/Parking_space#Marks_and_sp
ace_size

36

http://www.nature.com/nature/journal/v438/n7070/full/43
8900a.html. Like a handful of other publishers, *Nature* is
massively proprietary about their research. As such, this
article is available only on pay-per-view at $18 per article.
While you can try finding a free version online, you probably
shouldn't hold your breath. Like their evil cousin Elsevier (the
billion dollar Dutch academic publishing conglomerate),
Nature is pretty heavy duty in the fees department, even for
libraries. Their library price is so high you won't be able to find
it online, reinforcing the old adage – if you have to ask, you
can't afford it. But you will find references to Nature's 2010
rate hike at 400% - a jump that the University of California

system claimed would raise their subscription cost to a million dollars a year.

37

http://www.nh.gov/disability/information/architectural/documents/design_standards_parking.pdf

38

http://timeuseinstitute.org/Grocery%20White%20Paper%20 2008.pdf

39 http://www.thewalkingsite.com/10000steps.html

40 http://www.amazon.com/Miracle-Mindfulness-Introduction-Practice-Meditation-ebook/dp/B009U9S6VM

41

http://www.madonnahouse.org/restoration/2006/09/even_washing_dishes.html

42 http://www.washit.com/yearly-cost-savings/

43 http://housekeeping.about.com/od/laundry/f/fullload.htm

44 http://www.amazon.com/gp/product/B013XBVCKE

[45] http://www.foodprotection.org/files/food-protection-trends/Sep-Oct-14-Gerba.pdf

[46] https://www.bladderandbowelfoundation.org/bladder/bladder-conditions-and-symptoms/frequency/

[47] http://www.marketwatch.com/story/when-selling-hardwood-floor-beats-carpet-2014-06-02

[48] http://info.ekony.com/blog/benefits-of-wood-floors-for-real-estate

[49] http://www.pottytrainingconcepts.com/Tinkle-Targets-Cons.html

[50] http://www.statisticbrain.com/gym-membership-statistics/

[51] http://www.ywcagettysburg.org/special-events/sports-races/spirit-of-gettysburg-5k/

[52] https://runsignup.com/Race/PA/Biglerville/TheHardCiderRunGettysburg

53 http://www.halfmarathons.net/pennsylvania-gettysburg-blue-gray-half-marathon-5k/

54 http://www.gara-recpark.info/

55 http://paulssible5k.wix.com/paulssible5k#!about-us/c1e60

56 http://www.tuxedotrot.com/

57 http://www.pittsburghzoo.org/

58 http://www.runwildatlvzoo5k.com/

59 http://www.detroitzoo.org/Events/run-wild

60 http://www.milwaukeezoo.org/events/samson.php

61 http://www.milwaukeezoo.org/events/samson.php

62 http://www.czs.org/zoorunrun

63 http://www.zoomiami.org/Run

64 http://cincinnatizoo.org/events/

65 http://www.heartwalk.org/

[66] http://www.arthritis.org/get-involved/walk-to-cure-arthritis

[67] http://www.alz.org/

[68] http://namiwalks.org/

[69] http://www3.parkinson.org/site/PageServer?pagename=moving_day_cause_page

[70] http://donate.kidney.org/site/PageNavigator/kidney_walk_splash.html

[71] http://web.alsa.org/site/PageServer?pagename=WLK_landing#.VdXhS_lViko

[72] http://www.milwaukeezoo.org/events/samson.php

[73] http://www.resqwalk.com/

[74] http://www.wooftrax.com/

[75] http://www.charitymiles.org/

[76] https://soles4souls.org/

www.ingramcontent.com/pod-product-compliance
Lightning Source LLC
Chambersburg PA
CBHW072014290526
45787CB00013B/908